TH
NO POINT
WEIGHT LOSS
COOKBOOK

365 Days of Wholesome, Guilt-Free Eating

PARISH T. HARRIS

TABLE OF CONTENTS

Chapter 1

Breakfast Recipes

Scrambled eggs with spinach and feta

- Serving Size: This dish feeds 2 people.

- Cooking Time: Approximately 15 minutes.

- Prep Time: Around 5 minutes.

Nutrition Information:
- Calories: 210 per serving
- Fat: 15g
- Carbohydrates: 4g
- Protein: 15g

Ingredients:
- 4 big eggs
- 1 cup fresh spinach leaves, chopped
- 1/4 cup crumbled feta cheese
- 1 tablespoon olive oil
- Salt and pepper to taste

Directions:

1. In a medium-sized dish, break the eggs and whisk them until thoroughly blended. Set aside.

2. Heat the olive oil in a non-stick skillet over medium heat.

3. Add the chopped spinach to the pan and sauté for 1-2 minutes until wilted.

4. Pour the whisked eggs into the pan with the spinach.

5. Using a spatula, gently scramble the eggs, stirring regularly to achieve equal cooking. This procedure should take roughly 3-4 minutes.

6. Once the eggs are nearly set, sprinkle the crumbled feta cheese evenly over the top.

7. Continue cooking for another minute or until the eggs are totally set and the feta has slightly melted.

8. Season with salt and pepper according to your taste preferences.

9. Remove the pan from the heat and transfer the scrambled eggs to a serving plate.

10. Serve the scrambled eggs with spinach and feta immediately, while still hot.

Gluten-free oatmeal with blueberries and almond butter

- Serving Size: This dish makes roughly 2 servings.

- Cooking Time: The overall cooking time for this gluten-free oatmeal is roughly 15 minutes.

- Prep Time: The preparation time for this meal is roughly 5 minutes.

Nutrition Information:
- Calories: 350
- Total Fat: 15g
- Saturated Fat: 2g
- Cholesterol: 0mg
- Sodium: 60mg
- Total Carbohydrates: 46g
- Dietary Fiber: 8g
- Sugars: 10g
- Protein: 10g

Ingredients:
- 1 cup gluten-free rolled oats
- 2 cups water or dairy-free milk (such as almond milk or oat milk)
- 1/4 teaspoon salt
- 1/2 teaspoon cinnamon (optional)
- 1/2 cup fresh or frozen blueberries
- 2 tbsp almond butter

- Honey or maple syrup (optional, for sweetness)

Directions:
1. In a medium-sized saucepan, mix the gluten-free rolled oats, water or dairy-free milk, salt, and cinnamon (if wanted). Stir thoroughly.

2. Place the pot over medium heat and bring the mixture to a moderate boil. Reduce the heat to low and simmer for approximately 10 minutes, stirring periodically.

3. Add the blueberries to the oats and continue to simmer for a further 3-5 minutes, or until the blueberries are mushy and cooked through.

4. Remove the skillet from the heat and mix in the almond butter until fully incorporated.

5. Taste the oats and add honey or maple syrup if preferred, for added sweetness.

6. Allow the oatmeal to cool for a few minutes before serving to thicken slightly.

7. Divide the gluten-free oats into bowls and top with more blueberries and a dab of almond butter, if preferred.

Smoked salmon and avocado on rice cakes

- Serving Size: This dish makes roughly 4 servings.
- Cooking Time:
- Preparation time: 10 minutes
- Cooking time: 5 minutes

Nutrition Information (per serving):
- Calories: 210
- Total Fat: 10g
- Saturated Fat: 2g
- Cholesterol: 15mg
- Sodium: 300mg
- Carbohydrates: 20g
- Fiber: 3g
- Protein: 10g

Ingredients:
- 4 rice cakes
- 4 ounces of smoked salmon
- 1 ripe avocado
- 1 tablespoon freshly squeezed lemon juice
- 1 tablespoon chopped fresh dill
- Salt and pepper to taste

Directions:
1. Start by making the avocado combination. Cut the avocado in half, remove the pit, and scoop out the flesh into a small dish. Mash the avocado with a fork until you obtain a smooth consistency.

2. Add the freshly squeezed lemon juice to the mashed avocado and stir thoroughly. The lemon juice not only provides taste but also keeps the avocado from browning.

3. Next, add in the chopped fresh dill and season with salt and pepper according to your taste. Mix everything until fully blended. Set aside.

4. Toast the rice cakes until they are lovely and crispy. You may use a toaster or a toaster oven for this stage.

5. Once the rice cakes are finished, put a liberal portion of the avocado mixture onto each rice cake, ensuring it covers the whole surface.

6. Now, it's time to add the star of the dish: smoked salmon. Place roughly 1 ounce of smoked salmon on top of each rice cake, gently pushing it down to attach to the avocado mixture.

7. To garnish, you may add a sprinkling of freshly chopped dill or any other herbs of your choosing.

Quinoa breakfast dish with mixed berries and coconut flakes

- Serving Size: This dish makes roughly 2 servings.

- Cooking Time: Total cooking time is around 25 minutes.

- Prep Time: Preparation time takes roughly 5 minutes.

Nutrition Information:
- Calories: Approximately 280 per serving
- Total Fat: 6g
- Carbohydrates: 47g
- Fiber: 8g
- Protein: 10g

Ingredients:
- 1 cup quinoa, washed
- 2 cups water
- 1 cup mixed berries (such as strawberries, blueberries, or raspberries)
- 2 teaspoons coconut flakes
- 1 tablespoon honey or maple syrup (optional)
- 1 teaspoon vanilla extract
- A pinch of salt

Directions:
1. In a medium-sized saucepan, add the rinsed quinoa, water, and a teaspoon of salt.

2. Bring the mixture to a boil over medium-high heat.

3. Reduce the heat to low, cover the pot, and simmer for 15 minutes or until the quinoa is soft and the water is absorbed.

4. Remove from heat and let it settle, covered, for 5 minutes.

Banana pancakes prepared using gluten-free flour

- Serving Size: This recipe yields roughly 6 medium-sized pancakes.

- Prep Time: 10 minutes

- Cooking Time: 15 minutes

Ingredients:
- 2 ripe bananas
- 2 eggs
- 1 cup gluten-free flour blend (e.g., rice flour, almond flour, or a pre-made gluten-free flour mix)
- 1/2 cup milk (dairy or non-dairy choices include almond or oat milk)
- 1 teaspoon baking powder
- 1/2 teaspoon vanilla extract
- 1/4 teaspoon salt
- Cooking oil or butter for coating the pan

Directions:

1. In a mixing basin, mash the ripe bananas with a fork until smooth.

2. Add the eggs to the mashed bananas and whisk them together until fully mixed.

3. Next, add the gluten-free flour, milk, baking powder, vanilla extract, and salt to the banana-egg combination. Stir well until a smooth batter develops. If the batter looks too thick, you may add a bit more milk to get a pourable consistency.

4. Heat a non-stick pan or griddle over medium heat and gently coat it with cooking oil or butter.

5. Pour roughly 1/4 cup of the batter onto the heating skillet for each pancake. Use the back of a spoon to spread the batter into a circular shape.

6. Cook the pancakes for approximately 2-3 minutes, or until little bubbles start to form on the surface.

7. Flip the pancakes using a spatula and cook for a further 1-2 minutes or until golden brown.

8. Transfer the cooked pancakes to a platter and cover them with a clean kitchen towel to keep them warm while you prepare the remaining batter.

9. Serve the gluten-free banana pancakes warm with your favorite toppings such as fresh fruits, maple syrup, honey, or a dollop of yogurt.

Nutrition Information (approximate values per serving):
- Calories: 180
- Carbohydrates: 29g
- Protein: 6g
- Fat: 5g
- Fiber: 3g
- Sugar: 9g
- Sodium: 280mg

Chia seed pudding with low-FODMAP fruits like kiwi and pineapple.

- Serving Size: 2 servings

- Cooking Time: 0 minutes (excluding chilling time)

- Prep Time: 5 minutes

Nutrition Information (per serving):
- Calories: 250
- Carbohydrates: 40g
- Protein: 6g
- Fat: 8g

- Fiber: 10g

Ingredients:
- 4 tbsp chia seeds
- 1 cup lactose-free or low-FODMAP milk (such as almond milk or lactose-free cow's milk)
- 1 tablespoon maple syrup (optional, for sweetness)
- 1 kiwi, peeled and diced
- 1/2 cup pineapple, chopped
- Fresh mint leaves for garnish (optional)

Directions:
1. In a mixing dish, add the chia seeds and low-FODMAP milk. Stir carefully to ensure the chia seeds are properly dispersed in the milk.

2. If desired, add maple syrup to sweeten the pudding. Adjust the sweetness according to your taste preferences.

3. Let the mixture settle for 5 minutes, stirring regularly to avoid clumping. This enables the chia seeds to absorb the liquid and thicken the pudding.

4. Once the pudding has thickened, divide it into two serving glasses or bowls.

5. Top each serving with chopped kiwi and pineapple. You may also stack the fruits in between the chia seed pudding layers for a visually pleasing appearance.

6. Cover the cups or bowls with plastic wrap or a cover and chill for at least 2 hours or overnight. This enables the flavors to mingle and the chia seeds to thoroughly absorb the liquid.

7. Before serving, garnish with fresh mint leaves for extra freshness and scent (optional).

Chapter 2

Appetizers and Snacks

Caprese Skewers

- Serving Size: 4 servings

- Prep Time: 15 minutes

- Cooking Time: 0 minutes

Nutrition Information (per serving):
- Calories: 110
- Fat: 8g
- Carbohydrates: 3g
- Protein: 7g
- Sodium: 190mg

Ingredients:
- 8 cherry tomatoes
- 8 little mozzarella balls (bocconcini)
- Fresh basil leaves
- Balsamic glaze (optional)
- Salt and pepper to taste
- Wooden skewers

Directions:

1. Begin by preparing the ingredients. Rinse the cherry tomatoes and basil leaves. Drain and pat them dry with a paper towel. Make sure the mozzarella balls are at room temperature.

2. Take a wooden skewer and start constructing the Caprese skewers. Slide a cherry tomato onto the skewer, followed by a basil leaf folded in half, and finally a mozzarella ball. Repeat this technique until you have used all the ingredients.

3. Once all the skewers are constructed, season them with salt and pepper to taste. This procedure intensifies the tastes and brings out the natural taste of the foods.

4. Arrange the Caprese skewers on a serving dish or a plate. You may position them in a single layer or stack them slightly, depending on your inclination.

5. Optional: Drizzle balsamic glaze over the skewers to give a tangy and sweet taste. The glazing suits the Caprese combo well.

6. Serve the Caprese skewers immediately and enjoy! They are best served fresh and at room temperature.

Guacamole with Rice Crackers

- Serving Size: This dish yields roughly 4 servings.

- Cooking Time: Total cooking time for guacamole with rice crackers is roughly 15 minutes.

- Preparation Time: Preparing this wonderful snack will take roughly 10 minutes.

Nutrition Information:
- Calories: 180
- Total Fat: 15g
- Saturated Fat: 2g
- Cholesterol: 0mg
- Sodium: 320mg
- Total Carbohydrates: 12g
- Dietary Fiber: 7g
- Sugars: 1g
- Protein: 3g
- Vitamin D: 0mcg
- Calcium: 16mg
- Iron: 1mg
- Potassium: 570mg

Ingredients:
- 2 ripe avocados
- 1 lime, juiced
- 1/4 cup red onion, finely chopped

- 1/4 cup cilantro, finely chopped
- 1 tiny jalapeño pepper, seeded and coarsely chopped (optional)
- 1 garlic clove, minced 1/2 teaspoon cumin
- Salt & pepper to taste For serving:
- Rice crackers (as desired)

Directions:

1. Cut the avocados in half lengthwise, remove the pits, and scoop out the meat into a basin.

2. Mash the avocados with a fork until desired consistency is obtained. Some love thick guacamole, while others like it smoother.

3. Squeeze the lime juice over the mashed avocados and mix well to incorporate. Lime juice not only provides tanginess but also helps keep the avocados from turning brown.

4. Add the finely chopped red onion, cilantro, jalapeño pepper (if using), minced garlic, cumin, salt, and pepper to the bowl. Mix vigorously until all the ingredients are properly integrated.

5. Taste the guacamole and adjust the flavor as per your desire. You may add extra lime juice, salt, or pepper to suit your taste.

6. Transfer the guacamole to a serving plate and top with a sprinkling of fresh cilantro leaves.

7. Serve the guacamole with rice crackers, which offer a gluten-free and crunchy basis for the dip. Enjoy the delicious mix of creamy guacamole and crispy crackers.

Chicken Lettuce Wraps

- Serving Size: This dish makes roughly 4 servings.

- Prep Time: The preparation time for chicken lettuce wraps is roughly 15 minutes.

- Cooking Time: The cooking time for this dish is roughly 15 minutes.

Nutrition Information (per serving):
- Calories: 260
- Total Fat: 12g
- Saturated Fat: 2g
- Cholesterol: 70mg
- Sodium: 630mg
- Carbohydrates: 13g
- Fiber: 3g
- Sugar: 5g
- Protein: 24g

Ingredients:
- 1 pound ground chicken
- 2 teaspoons vegetable oil
- 2 cloves garlic, minced
- 1 small onion, coarsely chopped
- 2 teaspoons soy sauce
- 1 tablespoon hoisin sauce
- 1 tablespoon oyster sauce
- 1 teaspoon sesame oil
- 1/2 teaspoon red pepper flakes (optional)

For the Sauce:
- 3 tablespoons soy sauce
- 1 tablespoon hoisin sauce
- 1 tablespoon rice vinegar
- 1 teaspoon honey

For the Lettuce Wraps:
- 1 head iceberg or butter lettuce
- 1/2 cup shredded carrots
- 1/2 cup chopped green onions
- 1/4 cup chopped fresh cilantro
- 1/4 cup chopped peanuts (optional)

Directions:
1. In a large skillet or wok, heat the vegetable oil over medium heat. Add the minced garlic and diced onion, sautéing for approximately 2 minutes until they become aromatic and slightly softened.

2. Increase the heat to medium-high and add the ground chicken to the skillet. Break up the chicken with a spatula and heat until it's no longer pink, for roughly 5-6 minutes.

3. In a small bowl, whisk together the soy sauce, hoisin sauce, oyster sauce, sesame oil, and red pepper flakes (if using). Pour the sauce mixture over the cooked chicken in the pan, swirling carefully to coat evenly. Allow the chicken to simmer for a further 2-3 minutes, ensuring it is properly cooked and well-infused with the flavors.

4. In a separate small dish, mix the soy sauce, hoisin sauce, rice vinegar, and honey to prepare the sauce for the lettuce wraps. Stir thoroughly to incorporate the ingredients.

5. Wash and separate the lettuce leaves, wiping them dry with a paper towel. Arrange the lettuce leaves on a dish or individual plates.

6. To assemble, drop a tablespoon of the cooked chicken mixture onto each lettuce leaf. Top with shredded carrots, chopped green onions, fresh cilantro, and chopped peanuts if preferred. Drizzle the sauce over the fillings.

7. Serve the chicken lettuce wraps immediately, enabling your family or friends to wrap the contents in the lettuce leaves and enjoy the exquisite taste.

Smoked Salmon Cucumber Bites

- Serving Size: This recipe yields roughly 16 smoked salmon cucumber nibbles.

- Cooking Time: Total cooking time is roughly 30 minutes.

- Prep Time: Preparation time takes roughly 15 minutes.

Nutrition Info:
- Calories: 30
- Protein: 3g Fat: 1g
- Carbohydrates: 2g
- Fiber: 0g
- Sugar: 1g
- Sodium: 150mg

Ingredients:
- 1 big English cucumber
- 4 ounces of smoked salmon
- 4 ounces of cream cheese
- 2 teaspoons of fresh dill, chopped
- 1 tablespoon of fresh lemon juice
- Salt and pepper to taste

Directions:

1. Begin by cleaning the cucumber well. Slice it into roughly ½-inch thick circles. Place the cucumber slices on a paper towel to absorb any excess moisture.

2. In a small bowl, mix the cream cheese, fresh dill, lemon juice, salt, and pepper. Mix vigorously until the ingredients are equally combined.

3. Take a cucumber slice and apply a little quantity of the cream cheese mixture on top, forming a thin layer.

4. Cut the smoked salmon into tiny pieces that will fit atop the cucumber slices. Place a piece of smoked salmon on each cucumber slice.

5. Repeat the procedure with the remaining cucumber slices, cream cheese mixture, and smoked salmon.

6. Once all the bits are done, garnish them with a sprig of fresh dill or a sprinkling of minced dill for extra presentation and taste.

7. Arrange the smoked salmon cucumber bits on a serving tray and chill for at least 15 minutes to enable the flavors to melt together.

Roasted Red Pepper Hummus with Carrot Sticks

- Serving Size: This dish makes roughly 4 servings.

- Prep Time: The preparation time for Roasted Red Pepper Hummus with Carrot Sticks is roughly 10 minutes.

- Cooking Time: Since this recipe largely involves mixing and chopping, there is no cooking time necessary.

Nutrition Information:
- Calories: 150
- Total Fat: 7g
- Saturated Fat: 1g
- Sodium: 300mg
- Carbohydrates: 18g
- Fiber: 5g
- Protein: 6g

Ingredients:
- 1 can (15 ounces) chickpeas (garbanzo beans), drained and rinsed
- 2 roasted red peppers (from a jar or handmade)
- 2 cloves of garlic, minced
- 2 tablespoons tahini (sesame paste)
- 2 teaspoons fresh lemon juice
- 1 tablespoon extra virgin olive oil
- 1/2 teaspoon ground cumin
- Salt and pepper to taste
- Fresh carrot sticks, for serving

Directions:

1. Start by draining and washing the chickpeas well. This step helps eliminate excess salt and enhances the hummus's texture.

2. In a food processor or blender, mix the chickpeas, roasted red peppers, minced garlic, tahini, lemon juice, extra virgin olive oil, ground cumin, salt, and pepper. Blend until the mixture becomes smooth and creamy.

3. Taste the hummus and adjust the spices according to your liking. You may add extra lemon juice, salt, or pepper to increase the taste.

4. Transfer the hummus to a serving dish, and top it with a drizzle of olive oil, a sprinkling of cumin, or chopped fresh herbs like parsley or cilantro.

5. Serve the Roasted Red Pepper Hummus with freshly sliced carrot sticks on the side. The natural sweetness and texture of the carrots complement the hummus nicely.

Bacon-Wrapped Shrimp

- Serving Size: 4 servings

- Cooking Time: 20 minutes

- Prep Time: 15 minutes

Nutrition Information (per serving):
- Calories: 210
- Total Fat: 15g
- Cholesterol: 120mg
- Sodium: 500mg
- Protein: 16g
- Carbohydrates: 1g
- Fiber: 0g

Ingredients:
- 16 big shrimp, peeled and deveined
- 8 pieces of bacon, sliced in half
- 2 tablespoons olive oil
- 2 tablespoons maple syrup
- 1 teaspoon smoked paprika
- 1/2 teaspoon garlic powder
- 1/2 teaspoon salt
- 1/4 teaspoon black pepper
- Wooden toothpicks

Directions:

1. Preheat the oven to 400°F (200°C) and line a baking sheet with aluminum foil or parchment paper.

2. In a small bowl, mix the olive oil, maple syrup, smoked paprika, garlic powder, salt, and black pepper to form a marinade.

3. Place the shrimp in a big basin and pour the marinade over them. Toss carefully to ensure all the shrimp are covered. Allow them to marinade for 10 minutes.

4. Take a half piece of bacon and wrap it around each shrimp, fastening it with a wooden toothpick. Repeat this procedure until all the shrimp are wrapped.

5. Arrange the bacon-wrapped shrimp on the prepared baking sheet, allowing space between each one to promote uniform cooking.

6. Place the baking sheet in the preheated oven and bake for 10-12 minutes or until the bacon gets crispy and the shrimp are cooked through. Flip the shrimp halfway through the cooking time to achieve equal browning.

7. Once done, remove the baking sheet from the oven and allow the bacon-wrapped shrimp cool for a few minutes.

8. Serve the bacon-wrapped shrimp warm as an appetizer or as part of a main dish. Remove the toothpicks before serving.

Chapter 3

Soups and Salads

Chicken and Rice Soup

- Serving Size: This dish feeds 4 people.

- Cooking Time: Approximately 40 minutes.

- Prep Time: Approximately 15 minutes.

Nutrition Information (per serving):
- Calories: 320
- Fat: 10g
- Carbohydrates: 30g
- Protein: 25g
- Fiber: 3g

Ingredients:
- 2 boneless, skinless chicken breasts
- 1 tablespoon olive oil
- 1 medium onion, diced
- 2 carrots, peeled and sliced
- 2 celery stalks, chopped
- 2 cloves of garlic, minced
- 6 cups chicken broth (low sodium)
- 1 cup cooked rice
- 1 teaspoon dried thyme

- Salt and pepper to taste
- Fresh parsley, chopped (for garnish)

Directions:

1. Begin by cooking the chicken breasts. Season them with salt and pepper, then heat the olive oil in a large saucepan or Dutch oven over medium-high heat. Add the chicken breasts and cook for approximately 5-7 minutes each side, until golden brown and cooked through. Remove the chicken from the pot and put aside to cool.

2. In the same saucepan, add the chopped onion, carrots, celery, and minced garlic. Sauté the veggies for approximately 5 minutes, until they begin to soften.

3. While the veggies are simmering, shred the cooked chicken into bite-sized pieces.

4. Add the chicken stock, shredded chicken, cooked rice, and dried thyme to the saucepan. Stir thoroughly to incorporate all the ingredients. Bring the soup to a boil, then decrease the heat to low and let it simmer for approximately 20-25 minutes to enable the flavors to melt together.

5. Season the soup with salt and pepper according to your taste preferences.

6. Once the soup is finished, spoon it into bowls and top with fresh chopped parsley for extra freshness and color.

Tomato and Basil Salad

- Serving Size: This dish makes roughly 4 servings.

- Cooking Time: There is no cooking required with this recipe. It can be made in just a few minutes.

- Prep Time: The preparation time for Tomato and Basil Salad is around 10 minutes.

Nutrition Information:
- Calories: 70
- Total Fat: 4g
- Saturated Fat: 0.5g
- Sodium: 90mg
- Carbohydrates: 8g
- Fiber: 2g
- Sugar: 4g
- Protein: 2g

Ingredients:
- 4 big tomatoes (ripe and firm)
- 1 tiny red onion

- 1 cup fresh basil leaves
- 2 tablespoons extra-virgin olive oil
- 1 tablespoon balsamic vinegar
- Salt and pepper to taste

Directions:

1. Wash the tomatoes and basil leaves well. Pat them dry with a paper towel.

2. Slice the tomatoes into rounds or wedges, depending on your liking. Place them in a big basin.

3. Thinly slice the red onion and put it into the dish with the tomatoes.

4. Tear the basil leaves into tiny pieces and add them to the dish as well.

5. Drizzle the extra-virgin olive oil and balsamic vinegar over the tomatoes, onions, and basil.

6. Gently mix the ingredients until they are thoroughly covered with the dressing.

7. Season the salad with salt and pepper to taste. Be cautious not to oversalt, as the flavors of the tomatoes and basil should show.

8. Allow the salad to settle for approximately 10 minutes to allow the flavors to mingle together.

9. Serve the Tomato and Basil Salad as a side dish or as a light dinner on its own. It combines nicely with grilled meats, sandwiches, or crusty bread.

Lentil Soup

- Serving Size: 4-6 servings

- Cooking Time: Approximately 1 hour

- Prep Time: 10 minutes

Nutrition Information (per serving):
- Calories: 250
- Fat: 5g
- Carbohydrates: 40g
- Fiber: 10g
- Protein: 15g

Ingredients:
- 1 cup dry lentils (green or brown), washed and drained
- 1 onion, finely chopped
- 2 carrots, peeled and sliced
- 2 celery stalks, chopped
- 3 cloves of garlic, minced
- 1 can (400g) chopped tomatoes
- 4 cups vegetable broth 1 teaspoon ground cumin 1 teaspoon ground coriander

- 1/2 teaspoon smoked paprika
- Salt and pepper to taste
- Fresh cilantro or parsley for garnish (optional)

Directions:

1. In a big saucepan, heat a tablespoon of olive oil over medium heat. Add the chopped onions, carrots, and celery. Sauté for approximately 5 minutes until the veggies soften and the onions become transparent.

2. Add the minced garlic, cumin, coriander, and smoked paprika. Stir well to incorporate and simmer for another minute to enable the spices to unleash their flavors.

3. Add the rinsed lentils, diced tomatoes (with the juice), and vegetable broth to the saucepan. Stir everything together and bring the mixture to a boil.

4. Once boiling, decrease the heat to low, cover the pot, and simmer for around 40-45 minutes or until the lentils are cooked. Stir periodically to avoid sticking.

5. Taste the soup and season with salt and pepper according to your desire. Adjust the seasoning as required.

6. For a thicker consistency, you may use an immersion blender to partly mix the soup, or take a piece of the soup, blend it in a blender or food processor, and then return it to the pot.

7. Serve the lentil soup hot in bowls. Garnish with fresh cilantro or parsley if preferred. It works beautifully with a piece of crusty bread or a side salad.

Greek Salad

- Serving Size: This dish feeds 4 people.

- Cooking Time: The cooking time for Greek salad is brief since it largely entails combining the ingredients. No cooking is necessary.

- Prep Time: The prep time for Greek salad is roughly 15 minutes.

Nutrition Information (per serving):
- Calories: 240
- Fat: 20g
- Carbohydrates: 12g
- Protein: 4g
- Fiber: 3g

Ingredients:
- 4 medium-sized tomatoes, diced 1 big cucumber, peeled and diced
- 1 red onion, finely sliced 1 green bell pepper, diced 1 cup Kalamata olives, pitted 1 cup feta cheese, crumbled
- 2 tablespoons extra-virgin olive oil

- 2 teaspoons red wine vinegar
- 1 teaspoon dried oregano
- Salt and pepper to taste
- Freshly cut parsley for garnish (optional)

Directions:
1. In a large salad bowl, add the chopped tomatoes, cucumber, red onion, green bell pepper, and Kalamata olives.

2. Gently mix the ingredients to spread them evenly.

3. Sprinkle the crumbled feta cheese over the salad mixture.

4. In a small bowl, mix the extra-virgin olive oil, red wine vinegar, dried oregano, salt, and pepper.

5. Drizzle the dressing over the salad, ensuring all the components are gently covered.

6. Toss the salad gently to mix the ingredients and spread the dressing.

7. Taste and adjust the seasoning if required.

8. Garnish with freshly cut parsley for extra freshness and appearance.

9. Serve immediately and enjoy the tastes of the Mediterranean.

Carrot Ginger Soup

- Serving Size: 4 servings

- Cooking Time: 25-30 minutes

- Preparation Time: 10 minutes

Nutrition Information (per serving):
- Calories: 180
- Total Fat: 5g
- Saturated Fat: 1g
- Cholesterol: 0mg
- Sodium: 600mg
- Total Carbohydrate: 32g
- Dietary Fiber: 7g
- Sugars: 12g
- Protein: 4g
- Vitamin A: 450% RDA
- Vitamin C: 20% RDA
- Iron: 8% RDA
- Calcium: 10% RDA

Ingredients:
- 1 pound (450g) carrots, peeled and diced
- 1 medium-sized onion, chopped 2 cloves garlic, minced
- 1 tablespoon fresh ginger, grated
- 4 cups vegetable or chicken broth
- 1 cup coconut milk (or ordinary milk)
- 2 tablespoons olive oil
- Salt and pepper to taste
- Fresh cilantro or parsley for garnish (optional)

Directions:
1. Heat olive oil in a big saucepan over medium heat. Add the chopped onions and sauté for 2-3 minutes until they turn transparent.

2. Add the minced garlic and grated ginger to the saucepan, and sauté for an additional minute until aromatic.

3. Add the chopped carrots to the saucepan and combine them with the onion, garlic, and ginger combination. Sauté the carrots for approximately 5 minutes, allowing them to soften somewhat.

4. Pour in the vegetable or chicken broth, ensuring that the carrots are well covered. Bring the mixture to a boil, then decrease the heat to low and let it simmer for approximately 15-20 minutes, or until the carrots are soft.

5. Remove the saucepan from the heat and allow the soup to cool slightly. Use an immersion blender or transfer the liquid to a blender in stages to purée until smooth. If using a blender, be cautious as the heated liquid might expand.

6. Return the pureed soup to the stove and mix in the coconut milk (or normal milk) until fully blended. Season with salt and pepper to taste.

7. Place the saucepan back on the burner over low heat and reheat the soup for an additional 2-3 minutes.

8. Once warm, remove the saucepan from the burner. Ladle the Carrot Ginger Soup into dishes and garnish with fresh cilantro or parsley, if preferred.

Spinach and Strawberry Salad

- Serving Size: 4 servings

- Cooking Time: None

- Prep Time: 15 minutes

Nutrition Information (per serving):
- Calories: 120
- Total Fat: 5g
- Cholesterol: 0mg

- Sodium: 120mg
- Total Carbohydrate: 16g
- Dietary Fiber: 4g
- Sugars: 10g
- Protein: 5g
- Vitamin A: 70% RDA
- Vitamin C: 80% RDA
- Calcium: 10% RDA
- Iron: 15% RDA

Ingredients:
- 6 cups fresh spinach leaves, cleaned and dried
- 1 cup fresh strawberries, hulled and sliced
- 1/4 cup sliced almonds
- 1/4 cup crumbled feta cheese (optional)
- 2 tablespoons balsamic vinegar
- 1 tablespoon extra virgin olive oil
- 1 tablespoon honey
- Salt and pepper to taste

Directions:
1. In a large salad bowl, add the spinach leaves, sliced strawberries, sliced almonds, and crumbled feta cheese (if using). Toss lightly to mix.

2. In a small bowl, mix the balsamic vinegar, extra virgin olive oil, honey, salt, and pepper until thoroughly combined. This will act as the dressing for your salad.

3. Drizzle the dressing over the salad mixture and toss gently to coat all the ingredients equally.

4. Taste the salad and adjust the spices or dressing according to your desire.

5. Once the salad is made to your preference, serve it immediately and enjoy its refreshing flavors and textures.

Chapter 4

Main Dishes

Grilled chicken with roasted veggies

- Serving Size: 4 servings

- Cooking Time: 25-30 minutes

- Prep Time: 15 minutes

Nutrition Information (per serving):
- Calories: Approximately 350-400 calories
- Protein: 30-35 grams
- Fat: 10-12 grams
- Carbohydrates: 30-35 grams
- Fiber: 6-8 grams

Ingredients:
- 4 boneless, skinless chicken breasts
- 2 tablespoons olive oil
- 2 cloves garlic, minced
- 1 teaspoon paprika
- 1 teaspoon dried oregano
- Salt and pepper to taste
- 2 bell peppers (red, yellow, or orange), sliced 1 zucchini, sliced 1 red onion, sliced 1 cup cherry tomatoes
- Fresh herbs for garnish (optional)

Directions:

1. Preheat your grill to medium-high heat and preheat your oven to 400°F (200°C).

2. In a small bowl, mix the olive oil, minced garlic, paprika, dried oregano, salt, and pepper. Mix thoroughly to produce a marinade.

3. Place the chicken breasts in a shallow dish and pour the marinade over them, ensuring each piece is covered equally. Allow the chicken to marinade for 10-15 minutes.

4. While the chicken is marinating, prepare the veggies. Toss the sliced bell peppers, zucchini, red onion, and cherry tomatoes with a splash of olive oil, salt, and pepper.

5. Place the marinated chicken breasts on the hot grill and cook for approximately 6-8 minutes on each side, or until the internal temperature reaches 165°F (74°C). Cooking time may vary based on the thickness of the chicken breasts.

6. While the chicken is cooking, put the seasoned veggies on a baking sheet lined with parchment paper. Roast them in the preheated oven for around 15-20 minutes, or until they are soft and slightly caramelized.

7. Once the chicken is cooked through, take it from the grill and let it rest for a few minutes before slicing.

8. Serve the grilled chicken with the roasted veggies. Garnish with fresh herbs, if preferred.

Baked salmon with lemon and dill

- Serving Size: This dish feeds roughly 4 people.

- Cooking Time: The overall cooking time necessary for this meal is roughly 25-30 minutes.

- Prep Time: The prep time for this dish is roughly 10 minutes.

Nutrition Information:
- Calories: 300-350 kcal
- Protein: 30-35 grams
- Fat: 15-20 grams
- Carbohydrates: 5-10 grams
- Fiber: 1-2 grams

Ingredients:
- 4 salmon fillets (approximately 6 ounces each)
- 2 lemons
- Fresh dill, chopped
- Salt and pepper to taste
- Olive oil

Directions:

1. Preheat the oven to 400°F (200°C) and prepare a baking sheet with parchment paper or foil for easy cleaning.

2. Place the salmon fillets on the prepared baking sheet. Squeeze the juice of one lemon equally over the fillets.

3. Season the salmon with salt, pepper, and chopped fresh dill. Be liberal with the dill since it gives a lovely taste to the meal.

4. Slice the second lemon into thin rounds and set them on top of each salmon fillet. The lemon segments will infuse the fish with more zesty deliciousness.

5. Drizzle a tiny quantity of olive oil over each fillet to keep the salmon wet and prevent it from sticking to the baking sheet.

6. Bake the salmon in the preheated oven for approximately 15-20 minutes or until it is cooked through and flakes readily with a fork. Cooking durations may vary depending on the thickness of the fillets, so keep a watch on them to prevent overcooking.

7. Once the salmon is done, take it from the oven and let it rest for a few minutes before serving. This enables the flavors to mix and assures a delicate, juicy fish.

8. Serve the baked salmon with lemon and dill with your favorite side dishes such as roasted vegetables, steamed rice, or a fresh green salad.

Quinoa and veggie stir-fry

- Serving Size: 4 servings

- Cooking Time: 20 minutes

- Prep Time: 10 minutes

Nutrition Information (per serving):
- Calories: 300
- Carbohydrates: 50g
- Protein: 10g
- Fat: 8g
- Fiber: 7g

Ingredients:
- 1 cup quinoa, washed
- 2 cups water
- 2 tablespoons olive oil
- 1 small onion, finely sliced
- 2 garlic cloves, minced 1 red bell pepper, sliced 1 yellow bell pepper, sliced 1 zucchini, sliced 1 cup snap peas, trimmed
- 1 cup broccoli florets

- 2 tablespoons soy sauce (or tamari for a gluten-free alternative)
- 1 tablespoon sesame oil
- 1 tablespoon rice vinegar
- Salt and pepper to taste
- Sesame seeds (optional, for garnish)
- Fresh cilantro or parsley (optional, for garnish)

Directions:
1. In a medium-sized saucepan, mix the rinsed quinoa and water. Bring to a boil, then decrease the heat to low, cover, and simmer for approximately 15 minutes or until the quinoa is cooked and the water is absorbed. Set aside.

2. Heat olive oil in a large pan or wok over medium-high heat. Add the chopped onion and minced garlic, sautéing until they turn aromatic and faintly browned.

3. Add the sliced bell peppers, zucchini, snap peas, and broccoli florets to the pan. Stir-fry the veggies for around 5-7 minutes until they are crisp-tender but still maintain their beautiful colors.

4. In a small bowl, mix the soy sauce, sesame oil, and rice vinegar. Pour the sauce over the veggies in the pan, swirling carefully to cover them evenly.

5. Add the cooked quinoa to the pan and mix it with the veggies and sauce. Continue to simmer for a further 2-3

minutes, allowing the flavors to melt together. Season with salt and pepper to taste.

6. Remove the pan from heat and top with sesame seeds, fresh cilantro, or parsley for an added touch of flavor and appearance.

7. Serve the quinoa and veggie stir-fry hot and have a nutritious and tasty supper!

Turkey meatballs with zucchini noodles

- Serving Size: 4 servings

- Cooking Time: 25-30 minutes

- Prep Time: 15 minutes

Nutrition Information (per serving):
- Calories: 250
- Total Fat: 12g
- Carbohydrates: 10g
- Protein: 25g
- Fiber: 3g
- Sodium: 450mg

Ingredients:
- 1 pound ground turkey
- 1/2 cup breadcrumbs
- 1/4 cup grated Parmesan cheese 1/4 cup chopped fresh parsley
- 1/4 cup finely chopped onion
- 2 cloves garlic, minced 1 egg, beaten
- 1 teaspoon dried oregano
- 1/2 teaspoon salt
- 1/4 teaspoon black pepper

For the zucchini noodles:
- 4 medium-sized zucchinis
- 2 tablespoons olive oil
- Salt and pepper to taste
- For the sauce:
- 1 can (14 ounces) chopped tomatoes
- 2 cloves garlic, minced
- 1 teaspoon dried basil
- 1/2 teaspoon dried oregano
- Salt and pepper to taste

Directions:
1. Preheat your oven to 375°F (190°C) and line a baking sheet with parchment paper.

2. In a large mixing bowl, combine all the meatball ingredients: ground turkey, breadcrumbs, Parmesan cheese, parsley, onion, garlic, egg, dried oregano, salt,

and black pepper. Mix thoroughly until all the ingredients are equally combined.

3. Shape the turkey mixture into golf ball-sized meatballs, approximately 1.5 inches in diameter, and set them on the prepared baking sheet.

4. Bake the meatballs in the preheated oven for 15-20 minutes or until they are cooked through and lightly browned.

5. While the meatballs are baking, make the zucchini noodles. Using a spiralizer or a vegetable peeler, construct long, thin strands of zucchini noodles. If using a vegetable peeler, just slice the zucchini lengthwise into thin strips like noodles.

6. Heat olive oil in a large pan over medium heat. Add the minced garlic and sauté for approximately 1 minute until fragrant. Then add the chopped tomatoes, dried basil, dry oregano, salt, and pepper. Cook the sauce for approximately 5 minutes, allowing the flavors to meld together.

7. Once the meatballs are done, return them to the tomato sauce and gently boil for an additional 5 minutes.

8. In a second pan, heat another tablespoon of olive oil over medium heat. Add the zucchini noodles and sauté for 2-3 minutes until they become somewhat soft but still

have a crisp texture. Season with salt and pepper to taste.

Spicy shrimp and bell pepper skewers

- Serving Size: This dish feeds 4 people.

- Cooking Time: Approximately 10-12 minutes.

- Prep Time: Approximately 20 minutes.

Nutrition Info (per serving):
- Calories: 210
- Fat: 9g
- Carbohydrates: 9g
- Protein: 22g
- Fiber: 2g

Ingredients:
- 1 pound big shrimp, peeled and deveined
- 2 bell peppers (red, yellow, or orange), sliced into bits
- 1 tablespoon olive oil
- 1 tablespoon fresh lemon juice
- 2 cloves garlic, minced
- 1 teaspoon paprika
- 1/2 teaspoon cayenne pepper (modify to your spice level)
- Salt and pepper to taste

- Wooden or metal skewers

Directions:
1. Preheat your grill to medium-high heat. If using wooden skewers, soak them in water for 15 minutes to avoid scorching.

2. In a bowl, mix the olive oil, lemon juice, minced garlic, paprika, cayenne pepper, salt, and pepper. Mix thoroughly to produce a marinade.

3. Add the shrimp to the marinade and toss until they are equally covered. Allow the shrimp to marinade for approximately 10 minutes, while you prepare the bell peppers.

4. Thread the marinated shrimp and bell pepper pieces onto the skewers, alternating between shrimp and bell peppers.

5. Place the skewers on the hot grill and cook for approximately 5-6 minutes on each side or until the shrimp becomes pink and opaque. Be cautious not to overcook the shrimp, as they might turn rubbery.

6. Once the shrimp are done, take the skewers from the grill and let them rest for a couple of minutes.

7. Serve the spicy shrimp and bell pepper skewers hot, topped with a squeeze of fresh lemon juice and a sprinkling of chopped cilantro or parsley, if preferred.

Beef with broccoli stir-fry

- Serving Size: This dish feeds 4 people.

- Cooking Time: The cooking time for this beef and broccoli stir-fry is roughly 20 minutes.

- Prep Time: The prep time for this dish is roughly 10 minutes.

Nutrition Information:
- Calories: 250-300 per serving
- Total Fat: 10-12g
- Protein: 25-30g
- Carbohydrates: 15-20g
- Fiber: 3-5g

Ingredients:
- 1 lb (450g) flank steak or sirloin steak, thinly sliced
- 3 cups broccoli florets
- 2 tablespoons vegetable oil (divided)
- 3 cloves garlic, minced
- 1 teaspoon grated ginger
- 1/4 cup low-sodium soy sauce
- 2 tablespoons oyster sauce
- 1 tablespoon cornstarch
- 1/4 cup water
- Optional: red pepper flakes or sesame seeds for garnish

Directions:
1. In a small bowl, mix the soy sauce, oyster sauce, cornstarch, and water. Set the sauce aside.

2. Heat one tablespoon of vegetable oil in a large pan or wok over medium-high heat. Add the sliced meat and stir-fry for 2-3 minutes until browned. Remove the steak from the skillet and put it aside.

3. In the same skillet, add another tablespoon of vegetable oil. Add the minced garlic and grated ginger, and stir-fry for approximately 30 seconds until aromatic.

4. Add the broccoli florets to the pan and stir-fry for 3-4 minutes until they are brilliant green and slightly soft.

5. Return the cooked meat to the pan with the broccoli. Pour the sauce mixture over the meat and broccoli. Stir everything together until the sauce uniformly covers the ingredients.

6. Cook for a further 1-2 minutes until the sauce thickens and the meat is cooked to your preferred degree of doneness.

7. Remove the skillet from heat. Garnish with red pepper flakes or sesame seeds if preferred.

8. Serve the beef and broccoli stir-fry over steamed rice or noodles for a full supper.

Chapter 5

Sides and Accompaniments

Grilled chicken with roasted carrots

- Serving Size: 4 servings

- Cooking Time: 25-30 minutes

- Prep Time: 15 minutes

Nutrition Information (per serving):
- Calories: 300
- Protein: 30g
- Fat: 10g
- Carbohydrates: 25g
- Fiber: 6g

Ingredients:
- 4 boneless, skinless chicken breasts
- 1 pound carrots, peeled and sliced into thick slices
- 2 tablespoons olive oil
- 2 cloves garlic, minced
- 1 teaspoon dried thyme
- 1 teaspoon paprika
- Salt & pepper, to taste
- Fresh parsley, for garnish

Directions:

1. Preheat the grill to medium-high heat and preheat the oven to 425°F (220°C).

2. In a small bowl, mix the olive oil, minced garlic, dried thyme, paprika, salt, and pepper. Mix thoroughly to produce a marinade.

3. Place the chicken breasts in a shallow dish and pour the marinade over them. Make sure the chicken is fully coated. Allow it to marinade for at least 10 minutes or fridge for up to 2 hours for improved taste.

4. Meanwhile, in a separate dish, mix the carrot slices with a tablespoon of olive oil, salt, and pepper. Spread them evenly on a baking sheet.

5. Place the baking sheet with the carrots in the preheated oven. Roast for approximately 20-25 minutes or until the carrots are soft and slightly browned. Stir them once halfway through cooking for even browning.

6. While the carrots are roasting, take the chicken from the marinade and brush off any excess. Discard the leftover marinade.

7. Place the chicken breasts on the prepared grill. Cook for about 6-8 minutes each side or until the internal temperature reaches 165°F (74°C). Cooking time may vary based on the thickness of the chicken breasts.

8. Once the chicken is done, take it from the grill and let it rest for a few minutes. This enables the liquids to disperse and assures tender and juicy chicken.

9. Serve the grilled chicken with the roasted carrots. Garnish with fresh parsley for extra freshness and color.

Baked salmon with steamed green beans

- Serving Size: This dish feeds 4 people.

- Cooking Time: Approximately 25-30 minutes.

- Prep Time: Around 10-15 minutes.

Nutrition Information:
- Calories: 350-400 calories per serving
- Protein: 30-35 grams per serving
- Fat: 20-25 grams per serving
- Carbohydrates: 10-15 grams per serving
- Fiber: 4-6 grams per serving

Ingredients:
- 4 salmon fillets (approximately 6 ounces each), skin-on 1 pound fresh green beans, trimmed 2 tablespoons olive oil
- 2 cloves garlic, minced 1 lemon, sliced
- Salt and pepper to taste

- Optional: Fresh herbs such as dill or parsley for garnish

Directions:

1. Preheat the oven to 400°F (200°C).

2. Prepare the salmon fillets by washing them under cold water and wiping them dry with a paper towel. Season both sides of the fillets with salt and pepper according to your taste.

3. In a large baking dish, sprinkle 1 tablespoon of olive oil. Place the seasoned salmon fillets in the dish, skin-side down. Distribute the minced garlic equally over the fillets and sprinkle a couple of lemon slices on top for extra flavor.

4. Place the baking dish with the salmon in the preheated oven and bake for approximately 15-20 minutes, or until the salmon is cooked through and flakes easily with a fork. Cooking time may vary depending on the thickness of the fillets.

5. While the salmon is baking, cook the green beans. Fill a saucepan with approximately an inch of water and bring it to a boil. Place a steamer basket or colander over the boiling water and add the trimmed green beans. Cover and steam for about 5-7 minutes, or until the beans are soft but still crunchy.

6. Once the salmon is done, take it from the oven and let it rest for a couple of minutes. Meanwhile, sprinkle the

remaining tablespoon of olive oil over the cooked green beans and season with salt and pepper to taste.

7. Serve the baked salmon fillets with the steamed green beans. Garnish with fresh herbs, if preferred. Squeeze some lemon juice over the fish and beans for extra brightness.

Quinoa salad with cucumber and tomatoes

- Serving Size: This dish feeds 4 people.

- Cooking Time: The cooking time for this quinoa salad is roughly 15-20 minutes.

- Prep Time: The prep time for this dish is roughly 10-15 minutes.

Nutrition Information:
- Calories: 250
- Protein: 8g
- Fat: 10g
- Carbohydrates: 35g
- Fiber: 7g
- Sugar: 4g
- Sodium: 200mg

Ingredients:
- 1 cup quinoa
- 2 cups water
- 1 cucumber, diced
- 1-pint cherry tomatoes, halved
- 1/4 cup red onion, finely chopped
- 1/4 cup fresh parsley, chopped
- 1/4 cup fresh mint, chopped
- Juice of 1 lemon
- 2 tablespoons olive oil
- Salt and pepper to taste

Directions:
1. Rinse the quinoa: Start by washing the quinoa under cold water to eliminate any bitterness. Drain well.

2. Cook the quinoa: In a medium-sized saucepan, bring 2 cups of water to a boil. Add the rinsed quinoa and decrease the heat to low. Cover and simmer for approximately 15 minutes, or until the quinoa is cooked and the water is absorbed. Once cooked, fluff the quinoa with a fork and let it cool.

3. Prepare the vegetables: In a large bowl, add the diced cucumber, halved cherry tomatoes, finely chopped red onion, fresh parsley, and fresh mint.

4. Dress the salad: In a separate small bowl, stir together the lemon juice, olive oil, salt, and pepper. Pour the

dressing over the vegetable mixture and toss lightly to incorporate.

5. Add the quinoa: Once the quinoa has cooled, add it to the vegetable mixture and gently toss everything together until thoroughly incorporated.

6. Serve and enjoy: Transfer the quinoa salad to a serving plate and sprinkle with more fresh herbs if desired. Serve it immediately and enjoy the colorful flavors of this healthful salad.

Stir-fried tofu with bell peppers and zucchini

- Serving Size: 2-3 servings

- Cooking Time: 15-20 minutes

- Preparation Time: 10 minutes

Nutrition Information (per serving):
- Calories: 250
- Protein: 15g
- Fat: 15g
- Carbohydrates: 15g
- Fiber: 5g

Ingredients:
- 1 block of firm tofu (approx. 14 ounces)
- 1 red bell pepper
- 1 yellow bell pepper
- 1 medium-sized zucchini
- 2 tablespoons soy sauce (or tamari for a gluten-free alternative)
- 1 tablespoon sesame oil
- 1 tablespoon cornstarch
- 2 cloves of garlic, minced
- 1-inch piece of ginger, grated
- 1 tablespoon vegetable oil
- Salt and pepper to taste
- Optional garnish: sesame seeds and chopped green onions

Directions:
1. Start by preparing the tofu. Drain the tofu and gently press it between paper towels or a clean kitchen towel to remove excess moisture. Cut the tofu into tiny cubes or rectangular pieces.

2. In a mixing bowl, combine the soy sauce, sesame oil, minced garlic, grated ginger, and cornstarch. Whisk the ingredients until completely blended to make a delicious marinade.

3. Place the tofu pieces in the marinade and gently toss to coat them evenly. Allow the tofu to marinate for 5-10 minutes to absorb the aromas.

4. While the tofu is marinating, prepare the veggies. Remove the stems, seeds, and white pith from the bell peppers, and cut them into thin strips. Slice the zucchini into thin rounds.

5. Heat a tablespoon of vegetable oil in a big pan or wok over medium-high heat. Once the oil is heated, add the marinated tofu to the pan, keeping any remaining marinade. Stir-fry the tofu for 5-6 minutes or until it gets golden brown and slightly crunchy.

6. Remove the tofu from the pan and put it aside. In the same pan, add the bell peppers and zucchini. Stir-fry the veggies for 3-4 minutes or until they are tender-crisp.

7. Return the tofu to the pan with the veggies and pour in the remaining marinade. Toss everything together and heat for a further 1-2 minutes to enable the flavors to mingle.

8. Season the stir-fry with salt and pepper to taste. Remove from heat.

9. Garnish the stir-fried tofu with sesame seeds and chopped green onions, if preferred.

10. Serve the stir-fried tofu with bell peppers and zucchini hot over steamed rice or noodles. Enjoy the delicious blend of tastes and textures!

Roasted pork tenderloin with sautéed spinach

- Serving Size: 4 servings

- Cooking Time: 25-30 minutes

- Prep Time: 15 minutes

Nutrition Information (per serving):
- Calories: 350
- Protein: 30g
- Carbohydrates: 5g
- Fat: 22g
- Cholesterol: 90mg
- Fiber: 3g

Ingredients:
- 1 pound pork tenderloin
- 2 tablespoons olive oil
- 2 cloves garlic, minced
- 1 teaspoon dried thyme
- 1 teaspoon paprika
- Salt and pepper to taste
- 8 cups fresh spinach leaves, cleaned and trimmed
- 1 tablespoon butter
- 1 lemon, juiced
- Optional: lemon slices for garnish

Directions:
1. Preheat the oven to 400°F (200°C).

2. In a small bowl, mix the minced garlic, dried thyme, paprika, salt, and pepper. Rub this mixture all over the pork tenderloin, ensuring it is uniformly covered.

3. Heat one tablespoon of olive oil in an oven-safe skillet over medium-high heat. Once the pan is heated, add the pork tenderloin and sear it on both sides until beautifully browned, approximately 2 minutes on each side.

4. Transfer the pan to the preheated oven and roast the pork for 20-25 minutes, or until the internal temperature reaches 145°F (63°C). Remove the pan from the oven and allow the pork to rest for 5 minutes before slicing.

5. While the pork is resting, make the sautéed spinach. Heat the remaining tablespoon of olive oil and butter in a large pan over medium heat. Add the spinach leaves and sauté until wilted, approximately 3-4 minutes. Squeeze fresh lemon juice over the spinach and season with salt and pepper to taste.

6. To serve, slice the roasted pork tenderloin into thick medallions. Place a big quantity of sautéed spinach on each dish and place the pork pieces on top. Garnish with lemon slices if desired.

Turkey meatballs with gluten-free spaghetti and tomato sauce

- Serving Size: This dish feeds 4 people.

- Cooking Time: Total cooking time is around 40 minutes.

- Prep Time: Preparation time is roughly 20 minutes.

Nutrition Information:
- Calories: 350 per serving
- Total Fat: 12g
- Saturated Fat: 3g
- Cholesterol: 80mg
- Sodium: 600mg
- Carbohydrates: 30g
- Fiber: 5g
- Sugars: 8g
- Protein: 30g

Ingredients: For the meatballs:
- 1 pound ground turkey
- 1/2 cup gluten-free bread crumbs
- 1/4 cup grated Parmesan cheese
- 1/4 cup finely chopped fresh parsley
- 1 egg, beaten 2 cloves garlic, minced
- 1/2 teaspoon dried oregano
- 1/2 teaspoon dried basil
- 1/2 teaspoon salt 1/4 teaspoon black pepper

For the tomato sauce:
- 2 tablespoons olive oil
- 1 onion, finely chopped
- 2 cloves garlic, minced
- 1 can (14 ounces) crushed tomatoes
- 1 can (6 ounces) tomato paste
- 1 teaspoon dried basil
- 1 teaspoon dried oregano
- Salt and pepper to taste

For serving:
- 8 ounces of gluten-free spaghetti of your choice
- Fresh basil leaves, for garnish (optional)
- Grated Parmesan cheese, for garnish (optional)

Directions:
1. In a large bowl, mix the ground turkey, gluten-free bread crumbs, grated Parmesan cheese, parsley, beaten egg, chopped garlic, dried oregano, dried basil, salt, and black pepper. Mix thoroughly until all the ingredients are equally combined.

2. Shape the ingredients into meatballs of your chosen size. You may use an ice cream scoop or your hands to create the meatballs.
3. Heat olive oil in a large pan over medium heat. Add the meatballs and heat until browned on both sides, rotating them gently to ensure equal cooking. Remove the meatballs from the pan and put them aside.

4. In the same skillet, add the diced onion and minced garlic. Sauté until the onion turns transparent and aromatic.

5. Add the crushed tomatoes, tomato paste, dried basil, dried oregano, salt, and pepper to the skillet. Stir thoroughly to incorporate all the ingredients.

6. Return the meatballs to the pan with the tomato sauce. Cover the pan and let it simmer on low heat for approximately 20-25 minutes, or until the meatballs are cooked through and the sauce has thickened.

7. While the meatballs are boiling, prepare the gluten-free pasta according to the package directions until al dente. Drain the pasta and keep it aside.

8. To serve, add a serving of gluten-free spaghetti to each dish. Top with meatballs and tomato sauce. Garnish with fresh basil leaves and grated Parmesan cheese, if preferred.

Chapter 6

Desserts

Strawberry and Banana Smoothie

- Serving Size: This dish makes roughly 2 servings.

- Cooking Time: No cooking needed.

- Prep Time: The preparation time for this smoothie is roughly 5 minutes.

Nutrition Information:
- Calories: 150
- Carbohydrates: 35g Protein: 3g
- Fat: 1g
- Fiber: 5g
- Vitamin C: 90% of the recommended daily intake
- Potassium: 10% of the required daily intake

Ingredients:
- 1 cup fresh or frozen strawberries
- 2 ripe bananas
- 1 cup milk (dairy or plant-based)
- 1/2 cup plain Greek yogurt
- 1 tablespoon honey (optional, for extra sweetness)
- Ice cubes (optional, for a cold smoothie)

Directions:

- Wash the strawberries well and remove the stems.

- Peel the bananas and chop them into smaller bits for easy mixing.

- In a blender, add the strawberries, bananas, milk, Greek yogurt, and honey (if wanted).

- If you want a cooler smoothie, add a handful of ice cubes.

- Blend all the ingredients on high speed until smooth and creamy.

- If the consistency is too thick, you may add a bit more milk and combine again.

- Taste the smoothie and adjust the sweetness by adding additional honey if required.

- Pour the smoothie into cups and serve immediately.

Dark Chocolate Brownies

- Serving Size: This recipe makes roughly 16 excellent dark chocolate brownies.

- Cooking Time: Total cooking time: 30-35 minutes

- Prep Time: Preparation time: 15 minutes

Nutrition Information (per serving):
- Calories: 210
- Total Fat: 12g
- Saturated Fat: 7g
- Cholesterol: 45mg
- Sodium: 80mg
- Carbohydrates: 24g
- Fiber: 2g
- Sugars: 17g
- Protein: 3g

Ingredients:
- 1 cup dark chocolate chips (60-70% cocoa)
- 1/2 cup unsalted butter
- 1 cup granulated sugar
- 2 big eggs
- 1 teaspoon vanilla extract
- 3/4 cup all-purpose flour
- 1/4 cup unsweetened cocoa powder
- 1/4 teaspoon salt Optional: 1/2 cup chopped nuts (walnuts or pecans)

Directions:
1. Preheat your oven to 350°F (175°C). Grease an 8x8-inch baking pan or line it with parchment paper.

2. In a microwave-safe dish, mix the dark chocolate chips and butter. Microwave in 30-second intervals, stirring in between, until the chocolate and butter are melted and smooth.

3. In a separate large basin, mix the granulated sugar, eggs, and vanilla extract until thoroughly incorporated.

4. Slowly pour the melted chocolate mixture into the sugar and egg mixture, whisking continually until smooth and absorbed.

5. In another dish, whisk together the all-purpose flour, cocoa powder, and salt. Gradually add the dry ingredients to the wet mixture, stirring until just mixed. Be cautious not to overmix.

6. If desired, fold in the chopped nuts for extra texture and taste.

7. Pour the brownie batter onto the prepared baking pan, spreading it evenly.

8. Bake in the preheated oven for 25-30 minutes, or until a toothpick inserted into the middle comes out with a few wet crumbs. Avoid overbaking for a fudgy texture.

9. Remove the pan from the oven and allow the brownies to cool fully before cutting into squares.

10. Serve the dark chocolate brownies as is or with a dusting of powdered sugar, a dollop of whipped cream, or a scoop of vanilla ice cream for an added indulgence.

Lemon Bars

- Serving Size: 9-12 bars

- Cooking Time: 35-40 minutes

- Prep Time: 15 minutes

Nutrition Info: (per serving, based on 9 servings)
- Calories: 250
- Total Fat: 14g
- Saturated Fat: 8g
- Cholesterol: 90mg
- Sodium: 115mg
- Total Carbohydrate: 29g
- Dietary Fiber: 0.5g
- Sugars: 18g
- Protein: 3g

Ingredients:
- 1 cup all-purpose flour
- 1/4 cup powdered sugar
- 1/2 cup unsalted butter, softened
- 1 1/4 cups granulated sugar
- 1/4 cup all-purpose flour
- 1/4 teaspoon salt 3 big eggs
- 1/2 cup freshly squeezed lemon juice (approximately 3-4 lemons)
- 1 tablespoon lemon zest

Directions:
1. Preheat your oven to 350°F (175°C) and line an 8x8-inch baking sheet with parchment paper or gently oil it.

2. In a mixing basin, combine the flour, powdered sugar, and softened butter for the crust. Use a fork or pastry cutter to combine the ingredients until they create a crumbly texture.

3. Press the crust mixture evenly into the bottom of the prepared baking pan. Make sure the crust is well-packed.

4. Bake the crust in the preheated oven for approximately 15 minutes or until it gets gently brown. Remove from the oven and put aside.

5. While the crust is baking, prepare the filling. In another basin, mix the granulated sugar, flour, and salt.

6. In a separate dish, whisk the eggs, lemon juice, and lemon zest until completely blended.

7. Pour the egg mixture into the dry ingredients and whisk until everything is fully combined.

8. Pour the filling mixture over the cooked crust, spreading it evenly.

9. Bake the lemon bars for another 20-25 minutes or until the filling is set and the sides are slightly brown.

10. Remove the pan from the oven and allow it to cool fully on a wire rack. Once cooled, refrigerate for at least 2 hours to enable the bars to firm up.

11. Once cooled, remove the lemon bars from the pan using the parchment paper or by carefully lifting the sides. Cut into squares or bars of your preferred size.

Coconut Macaroons

- Serving size: This recipe yields roughly 24 macaroons.

- Cooking time: 20-25 minutes

- Prep time: 15 minutes

Nutrition info: (Per serving = 1 macaroon)
- Calories: 100
- Total Fat: 7g
- Saturated Fat: 6g
- Cholesterol: 0mg
- Sodium: 50mg
- Total Carbohydrates: 9g
- Dietary Fiber: 1g
- Sugars: 7g
- Protein: 1g

Ingredients:
- 3 cups shredded coconut (sweetened or unsweetened)
- 3/4 cup sweetened condensed milk
- 2 big egg whites
- 1 teaspoon vanilla extract
- 1/4 teaspoon salt

Directions:
1. Preheat your oven to 325°F (160°C) and line a baking sheet with parchment paper.

2. In a mixing dish, add the shredded coconut, sweetened condensed milk, vanilla essence, and salt. Stir well until all the ingredients are equally blended.

3. In a separate dish, whip the egg whites until they form firm peaks. This may be done with an electric mixer or by whisking vigorously by hand.

4. Gently incorporate the beaten egg whites into the coconut mixture until well-mixed. Be cautious not to overmix; you want to keep the mixture light and airy.

5. Using a spoon or a cookie scoop, place rounded scoops of the mixture onto the prepared baking sheet, spreading them about an inch apart.

6. Bake the macaroons in the preheated oven for 20-25 minutes, or until they become golden brown on the edges.

7. Remove the baking sheet from the oven and allow the macaroons to cool on the sheet for a few minutes. Then move them to a wire rack to cool fully.

8. Once the macaroons have cooled, they are ready to be savored. Serve them as a lovely dessert or a sweet snack.

Raspberry Chia Pudding

- Serving Size: This dish makes roughly 2 servings.

- Cooking Time: The cooking time for raspberry chia pudding is roughly 10 minutes.

- Prep Time: The prep time for raspberry chia pudding is roughly 10 minutes. However, it needs an extra 4 hours for the pudding to set in the refrigerator.

Nutrition Information (per serving):
- Calories: 200
- Total Fat: 8g
- Saturated Fat: 1g
- Cholesterol: 0mg
- Sodium: 60mg
- Carbohydrates: 28g
- Fiber: 15g
- Sugars: 8g
- Protein: 6g
- Vitamin C: 35%
- Calcium: 20%
- Iron: 10%

Ingredients:
- 1 cup fresh or frozen raspberries
- 1 cup almond milk (or any other plant-based milk)
- 1/4 cup chia seeds
- 2 tablespoons honey or maple syrup (adjust to taste)

- 1/2 teaspoon vanilla extract
- Fresh raspberries and mint leaves (for garnish)

Directions:
1. In a blender, add the raspberries, almond milk, honey or maple syrup, and vanilla extract. Blend until smooth and fully integrated.
2. Pour the raspberry mixture into a dish or individual serving glasses.
3. Add the chia seeds to the raspberry mixture and swirl well to ensure they are equally distributed.
4. Cover the bowl or glasses with plastic wrap or a cover and chill for at least 4 hours or overnight. This causes the chia seeds to absorb the liquid and generate a pudding-like consistency.
5. After the pudding has set, give it a thorough stir to break up any clumps that may have formed.
6. Serve the raspberry chia pudding in separate dishes or glasses. Garnish with fresh raspberries and mint leaves for an additional touch.

Almond Butter Cookies

- Serving Size: Approximately 18 cookies

- Cooking Time: 12-15 minutes

- Prep Time: 15 minutes

Nutrition Info (per cookie):
- Calories: 150
- Fat: 11g
- Carbohydrates: 11g
- Protein: 4g
- Fiber: 2g
- Sugar: 7g

Ingredients:
- 1 cup almond butter (smooth or crunchy, depending on your desire)
- 1/2 cup coconut sugar (or any other granulated sweetener of your choosing)
- 1 big egg
- 1 teaspoon vanilla extract
- 1/2 teaspoon baking soda
- 1/4 teaspoon salt

Directions:
1. Preheat your oven to 350°F (175°C) and line a baking sheet with parchment paper.

2. In a mixing dish, combine the almond butter, coconut sugar, egg, vanilla extract, baking soda, and salt. Stir vigorously until all the components are integrated and the mixture is smooth.

3. Scoop out rounded teaspoons of dough and shape them into balls. Place them on the prepared baking sheet, allowing a little space between each cookie.

4. Use a fork to gently push down on each cookie ball, forming a crisscross pattern on the top.

5. Bake the cookies in the preheated oven for 12-15 minutes, or until the edges are slightly golden brown. Be cautious not to overcook them, since almond butter may burn rapidly.

6. Once cooked, remove the cookies from the oven and allow them to cool on the baking sheet for a few minutes. Then move them to a wire rack to cool fully.

7. Once chilled, the almond butter cookies are ready to be eaten! Store any leftovers in an airtight jar at room temperature for up to 5 days.

Made in United States
North Haven, CT
15 August 2024